SKINNY

RECIPES

Low calorie recipes for your favourite guilty pleasures

Table of Contents

Get your <u>Two</u> Free Bonuses

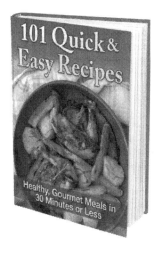

As a thank you, I want to give you this amazing collection of **101 Quick and Easy Recipes**, completely free of charge, as my gift to you. Download it now!

Click here to get it FREE!!

http://bit.ly/free101recipes

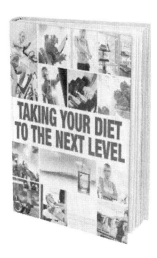

As a thank you, I want to give you this amazing report entitled **Taking Your Diet to the Next Level**, completely free of charge, as my gift to you. Download it now!

Click here to get it FREE!!

http://bit.ly/nextleveldiet

Introduction

If you are like everyone else, you want to improve your diet, be healthier and have tons of energy. There is just one problem, most health and diet food sucks. It's bland, dry and just doesn't taste very good. if you are like me, you go on a diet, eat healthy for a few days and then all you want is fried chicken and macaroni and cheese, and there goes the diet. But eventually I realized that a diet without good food will never be a diet I can follow for the long term.

So I found a little trick, and it's so simple and easy, you'll wonder why you didn't think of it.

You can eat all the foods you like, all the traditionally unhealthy and fatty foods that you love, just substitute some of the ingredients for healthier options. It's as simple as that.

With a few changes and substitutions to your regular cooking methods and ingredients, you can make a high calorie, high fat meal turn into a healthy, nutritious meal, that tastes great.

There is no need to change the whole recipe, all you have to do is pinpoint unhealthy ingredients and change them into healthier substitutes. For example, you can use greek yogurt instead of sour cream. You can even make amazingly tasty mashed cauliflower to replace your usual mashed potatoes or use more egg whites in place of cholesterol-rich whole eggs.

You can also opt to roast chicken in the oven rather than deep-frying them or steam vegetables instead of boiling them. There are so many ways to make traditionally guilty pleasures into healthy meals, all you have to do is read on, to learn how.

I hope you enjoy the book.

Classic Coleslaw

Greek Yogurt in; Mayonnaise out. Low-fat milk in; whole milk out.

Makes 6 servings

6 cups **cabbage**, finely shredded

1 small **onion**, grated

1 small **carrot**, grated

2 tsp. **salt**

DRESSING

1 cup Greek yogurt

4 tbsp. **sugar**

4 tbsp. apple cider vinegar

salt and pepper

1/2 cup fat-free milk

Into a colander, sprinkle cabbage with salt. Mix and let drain for about half an hour.

Meanwhile, into a large salad bowl, combine all ingredients for the dressing, whisk until smooth.

Mix dressing ingredients until smooth.

Squeeze cabbage to remove excess water and add into the bowl with the dressing. Mix in carrot and onions. Slowly mix to blend well. Cover with plastic wrap and chill for at least 2 hours.

Amount Per Serving: Calories 238.4; Calories from Fat 30; Total Fat 13.6 g; saturated Fat 2.1 g; Cholesterol 11.6 mg; Sodium 1092.4 mg; Total Carbohydrate 28.7 g; Dietary Fiber 3.8 g; Sugars 17.2 g; Protein 3.0 g

Baked Sweet Potato Fries

Sweet Potatoes in; Potatoes out

Makes 4 Servings

4 large **sweet potatoes**, peeled, and cut into 2-inch thick wedges

2 tbsp. olive oil

1 1/2 ground **cinnamon**

1 tsp. **salt**

1 tsp. pepper

3 tbsp. reduced-fat cheddar cheese, grated

Preheat oven to 350 ºF. Lightly grease a baking sheet.

Evenly spread sweet potatoes onto prepared baking sheet, Drizzle with olive oil, sprinkle with cinnamon, salt and pepper and bake for about 40 minutes or until golden and fork tender.

Take out from the oven and evenly sprinkle the cheese all over the top. Cool slightly on wire rack and serve on individual plates.

Amount Per Serving: Calories 415; Total Fat 30 g; saturated Fat 4 g; Sodium 94 mg; Total Carbohydrate 35 g; Dietary Fiber 6 g; Sugars 8 g; Protein 3.0 g

Low Fat Blue Berry Muffins

Almond and coconut flours in; All-purpose flour out.
Coconut sugar in; cane sugar out.

Makes 6 servings

1 cup almond flour flour

3/4 cup coconut flour

3/4 cup coconut sugar

1 tbsp. baking powder

1 tsp. **lemon zest**, finely shredded

3 egg **whites**

2/3 cup buttermilk

1/3 cup unsweetened applesauce

1 tsp. **vanilla**

1 cup fresh blueberries

Preheat oven to 400 ºF. Lightly grease a 6 cup muffin
pan.

Into a large bowl, combine flours with the rest of the dry
ingredients. Mix well.

Into another bowl, whisk egg whites until foamy. Mix in the buttermilk, vanilla and applesauce. Slowly add this mixture into the flour mixture. Mix until batter is formed. Add the berries, fold to combine.

Fill cups with batter, each 3/4 full and bake for about 23 minutes. Cool on wire rack and serve.

Amount Per Serving: Calories 262.8; Calories from Fat 784; Total Fat 0.8 g; Saturated Fat 0.2 g; Cholesterol 1.0 mg; Sodium 230.1 mg; Total Carbohydrate 58.8 g; Dietary Fiber 3.1 g; Sugars 28.9 g; Protein 6.5 g

Vegetable Salad with Cottage Cheese

Cottage Cheese in; Dairy cheese out. Salt out; lemon juice in.

Makes 2 serving

1/3 cup low fat **cottage cheese**

8 slices **cucumbers**, chopped

4 slices **tomatoes**, chopped

1 stalk **celery**, chopped

2 slices **red onion**, chopped

Dash of **lemon juice** (more if needed to make up for no salt)

Black pepper to taste

cabbage, lettuce, shredded

Into a bowl, combine all ingredients, toss to coat.

Serve topped with greens. Enjoy as is or stuffed as a sandwich filling.

Amount Per Serving: Calories 33.8; Calories from Fat 3; Total Fat 0.4 g; Saturated Fat 0.2 g; Cholesterol 1.1 mg; Sodium 75.3 mg; Total Carbohydrate 5.4 g; Dietary Fiber 1.1 g; Sugars 2.6 g; Protein 2.7 g

Caesar Salad with Avocado mash

Avocado mash takes the place of mayonnaise.

Makes 6 servings

6 cloves **garlic**, peeled, minced

3/4 cup **avocado**, mashed

1 tsp. Dijon mustard

5 anchovy fillets, minced

6 tbsp. **parmesan cheese**, finely grated, divided

1 tbsp. lemon juice

1 tsp. Worcestershire sauce

salt to taste

ground **black pepper** to taste

1/4 cup olive oil

4 cups **bread**, cubed

1 head **romaine lettuce**, torn into bite-size pieces

Into a bowl, combine avocado mash with anchovies, 2 tbsp. of the Parmesan cheese, mustard, Worcestershire sauce, and lemon juice. Mix well. Sprinkle with salt and black pepper to taste. Chill until ready to use.

Into a large pan, heat oil over medium heat Cook and stir garlic until browned. Remove garlic into a bowl. Place bread chunks into the hot oil and cook, turning repeatedly, until lightly browned. Remove bread into a plate; season with salt and pepper.

Into a large salad bowl, combine lettuce and avocado dressing along with remaining cheese, toasted garlic and bread cubes. Toss until fully blended.

Amount Per Serving: Calories 184; Total Fat 1.5 g; Saturated Fat 0.2 g; Cholesterol 18 mg; Sodium 549 mg; Total Carbohydrate 16.3 g; Dietary Fiber 1.8 g; Sugars 2.6 g; Protein 5.8 g

Chicken Pot Pie Soup

No crust, no butter, and no milk.

Makes 5 Servings

1 lb. boneless chicken breast

1 (10-oz.) can fat-free **cream of chicken soup**

4 cups low-sodium **chicken broth**

1 (16-oz.) frozen bag of peas, carrots, corn, and green beans

1 cup **potato,** peeled, diced

1/2 cup **onion,** diced

1 tsp. **thyme**

1 tsp. **pepper**

1 bay **leaf**

2 tbsp. corn starch

2 tbsp. **water**

Into a slow cooker, combine all ingredients, except corn starch and water. Mix, cover and cook on Low for about 8 hours or on High for about 5 hours.

Into a small bowl, dissolve corn starch in water. Mix into the dish, cook for a few minutes until thickened.

Amount Per Serving: Calories 293; Total Fat 12 g; Saturated Fat 3 g; Cholesterol 60 mg; Sodium 377 mg; Total Carbohydrate 23; Dietary Fiber 4 g; Sugars 5 g; Protein 25 g

Oatmeal Cookies

Whole oats instead of wheat flour

Makes 18 cookies

2 -2 1/2 cups **whole oats**

4 ripe **bananas**

1 tsp. baking soda

2 tbsp. **honey**

1 tbsp. **cinnamon** (to taste)

1/4 cup **almonds**, crushed

Preheat oven to 350 ºF.

Into a bowl, mash bananas until smooth. Mix in the rest of the ingredients, blend until batter is formed. Add more honey if it's too dry or more oats if too wet.

Scoop tablespoonful portions of the batter onto a baking sheet; pat slightly to flatten. Bake for about 17 minutes or until golden brown.

Amount Per Serving: Calories 98.8; Calories from Fat 11; Total Fat 1.2 g; Saturated Fat 0.2 ; Cholesterol 0.0 mg; Sodium 70.7 mg; Total Carbohydrate 19.7 g; Dietary Fiber 2.7 g; Sugars 5.1 g; Protein 3.2 g

Mashed Cauliflower

Potato out; Cauliflower in

Makes 4 servings

1 lb. **cauliflower**, cut into florets

1 tbsp. coconut milk

1 tbsp. **garlic** powder

1 tsp. **onion** powder

salt and ground **black pepper** to taste

Into a pot of boiling salted water, cook cauliflower for about 18 minutes or until tender. Drain into a colander and place back into the pot.

Pour in coconut milk and blend using an immersion blender until smooth. Mix in garlic powder, onion powder; sprinkle salt, and pepper to taste.

Amount Per Serving: Calories 47; Total Fat 1.0 g; Cholesterol 0.0 mg; Sodium 141 mg; Total Carbohydrate 8.7 g; Dietary Fiber 3.7 g; Protein 3.1 g

Mayonnaise-free Waldorf Salad

Mayonnaise out; Greek yogurt in

Makes 4 servings

1 large **apple**, cored, cubed

1/3 cup Greek yogurt

1 cup **walnuts**, shelled

1/2 cup **raisins**

1/2 cup cranberries

25 baby **carrots,** julienned

2 stalks **celery,** chopped

2 tbsp. lemon juice

1 tbsp. **sugar**

Into a bowl, drizzle lemon juice over the freshly cut apples, toss to evenly coat. Combine the rest of the ingredients, gently toss to blend.

Chill until ready to serve. Serve with your favourite cooked meat.

Amount Per Serving: Calories 317.2; Calories from Fat 174; Total Fat 19.3 g; Saturated Fat 1.8 g; Cholesterol 0.0

mg; Sodium 68.1 mg; Total Carbohydrate 36.6 g; Dietary Fiber 5.9 g; Sugars 24.1 g; Protein 5.7 g

Creamy Chicken Soup

Coconut milk in, whole milk out

Makes 4 servings

2 cups **coconut milk,** divided

2 **lemon grass**, chopped

4 slices piece **fresh ginger,** peeled

5 **lime leaves**, torn in half

3/4 lb. skinless, boneless **chicken breasts**, cut into strips

5 tbsp. fish sauce

2 tbsp. white sugar

1 cup coconut milk

1/2 cup lime juice

1 tsp. red curry paste

1/4 cup **cilantro,** coarsely chopped

15 **green chiles**, crushed

Into a large saucepan, combine 1 cup coconut milk, lemon grass, ginger, and lime leaves; bring to a boil over medium high heat. Add chicken, season with fish sauce and sugar, lower heat to medium and cook for another 5 minutes or until chicken is well cooked.

Pour in the remaining coconut milk and simmer for 3 minutes more. Serve in individual serving bowls, garnished with cilantro and green chiles.

Amount Per Serving: Calories 436; Calories from Fat 174; Total Fat 25.6 g; Saturated Fat 1.8 g; Cholesterol 49 mg; Sodium 1477 mg; Total Carbohydrate 32 g; Dietary Fiber 4.2 g; Sugars 24.1 g; Protein 26.7 g

Tomato-free Macaroni and Cheese

Tomatoes out, Butternut squash in.

Makes 8 servings

1 lb. elbow macaroni

2 (10-oz.) pack **butternut squash**, pureed

2 cups low-fat milk

2 cups **Cheddar cheese**, grated

1/2 cup part-skim **ricotta cheese**

1 tsp. **salt**

1 tsp. dried mustard powder

1/8 tsp. cayenne pepper

1/2 cup bread crumbs

3 tbsp. **Parmesan cheese**, grated

2 tbsp. olive oil

Preheat oven to 375 ºF. Lightly grease a 9 X 13-inch baking pan.

Into a pot of boiling salted water, cook macaroni for about 8 minutes or until al dente. Drain into a colander, rinse with running water and transfer into a bowl.

While the pasta is cooking, combine squash with milk into a saucepan and bring to a simmer over medium heat. Away from heat, add the cheeses, mustard, cayenne pepper and salt. Mix well to blend. Pour into the bowl with the macaroni. Mix to blend.

Spread pasta and cheese mixture into the prepared baking pan and bake for about 20 minutes. Increase heat to broiling and cook for another 3 minutes or until top is golden brown.

Amount Per Serving: Calories 618; Total Fat 29 g; Saturated Fat 16 g; Cholesterol 79 mg; Sodium 859 mg; Total Carbohydrate 60 g; Dietary Fiber 4.0 g; Sugars 7.0 g; Protein 30 g

Reuben Sandwiches

Lower Sodium, lower calorie and lower saturated fat

Makes 4 servings

Dressing:

1 tbsp. chili sauce

1 tsp. Worcestershire sauce

1/4 cup cholesterol-free canola mayonnaise

2 tsp. **dill pickle,** finely minced

1/2 tsp. **onion**, grated

Sandwiches:

8 (3/4-oz.) slices **rye bread**

3/4 cup **Swiss cheese,** shaved

4 oz. **corned beef**, low-sodium, thinly sliced

1 cup **sauerkraut**, organic, drained

Preheat oven to its broiling temperature.

Into a bowl, combine all the ingredients for the dressing, mix well to blend.

Arrange bread slices in a single layer on a baking sheet and toast for about 1 1/2 minutes or until browned. Flip sides and toast for another minute or until lightly browned.

Sprinkle cheese over lightly toasted slices and broil for about a minute or until cheese melts. Spread cheese-coated sides of bread slice with about 1 tablespoon of the dressing. Top each with an ounce of corned beef, and 1/4 cup sauerkraut. Put remaining bread slices on tops.

Amount Per Serving: Calories 336; Total Fat 20 g; Saturated Fat 5.6 g; Cholesterol 40 mg; Sodium 790 mg; Total Carbohydrate 24.2 g; Dietary Fiber 3.4 g; Iron 1.9mg; Sugars 7.0 g; Protein 14.7 g

Vegetable Lasagna

Pasta out, squash in

Makes 8 servings

1 (4.5 lbs.) large **spaghetti squash**

4 oz. goat cheese

15 oz. ricotta cheese

8 oz. mozzarella cheese, grated

1 whole **egg**

1/4 cup **parmesan cheese**, grated

5 cups **tomatoes**, chopped

1 lb. of turkey sausage

1 small **onion**, finely diced

4 large **garlic** cloves, minced

salt and pepper

2 tbsp. olive oil, divided

Preheat oven to 400 ºF.

Create pricks all over the squash, place on a baking dish and roast for about an hour or until fork tender. Set aside to cool.

Into a saucepan, heat 1 tbsp. olive oil over medium high heat, cook turkey sausage while mixing until they turn to browned pieces. Mix in onion and half of garlic and cook for about 4 minutes or until tender. Add tomatoes, mix, partially cover and cook for about 2 hours over low heat. Sprinkle salt and pepper to taste.

Meanwhile, cut into half the squash, take out seeds and scoop out flesh into a bowl. Set aside. Into another bowl, combine goat and parmesan cheeses, egg and half of the mozzarella. Set aside.

Into a clean saucepan, heat remaining oil over medium flame. Add remaining garlic and cook until lightly browned. Add squash and cook for about 3 minutes or until squash start to brown. Sprinkle salt and pepper to taste.

Lower oven temperature to 375 °F.

Into a baking dish, spread half of the turkey-tomato mixture; layer squash and top with the cheese mixture. Spread the remaining tomato sauce and drizzle top with remaining mozzarella. Bake for about an hour or until brown and bubbly.

Amount Per Serving: Calories 396.9; Calories from Fat 251; Total Fat 27.9 g; Saturated Fat 12.5 g; Cholesterol 117.9 mg; Sodium 890.3 mg; Total Carbohydrate 10.3 g; Dietary Fiber 0.7 g; Sugars 3.0 g; Protein 26.6 g

Mushroom Meat Loaf

Beef out; turkey and mushrooms in. Bread crumbs out; instant oats in.

Makes 8 servings

1 lb. cremini mushrooms

1 tbsp. coconut oil

6 **garlic** cloves, minced

1 1/4 cups **onion,** finely chopped

2 tbsp. dry sherry

2 tsp. **fresh thyme,** chopped

1/2 cup quick-cooking **instant oats**

5/8 tsp. kosher salt

1/2 tsp. black pepper

8 oz. ground turkey

1 whole **egg**, whisked

1/4 cup **ketchup**, low-sodium, divided

Preheat the oven to 375 °F. Lightly grease a 7 x 3 inch paper-lined baking dish.

Into a food processor, pulse half of the mushrooms until minced; transfer into a bowl. Clean the processor.

Into a pan, heat oil over medium-high flame and cook onions for about 3 minutes or until translucent. Mix in garlic, cook for about a minute. Add all the mushrooms and cook with stirring for about 7 minutes or until starting to brown. Pour in sherry and cook for another minute. Put off heat and stir in thyme. Set aside to cool a bit.

Into the prepared dish, mix mushroom-spice mixture with egg, oats, turkey, salt and pepper. Mix to blend. Flatten surface and bake for about 20 minutes. Take out and brush top with one-half of the ketchup and bake for another 15 minutes until inner part reaches 160°F.

Take out from oven; brush with ketchup and cut into slices.

Amount Per Serving: Calories 253; Fat 10.9 g; Saturated fat 3 g; Mono fat 5.2 g; Poly fat 1.5 g; Protein 17.9 g;

Carbohydrate 20.2 g; Fiber 2.1 g; Cholesterol 83 mg; Iron 2.3 mg; Sodium 389 mg; Calcium 59 mg

Vegetarian Chilli

Meat out; beans in.

Makes 6 servings

2 tbsp. extra-virgin **olive oil**

1/2 cup **red bell pepper**, chopped

1/2 cup **yellow onion**, chopped

1 **garlic clove**, roasted

1/2 cup **carrot**, grated

2 tbsp. **cumin seeds**, toasted

3 tbsp. chili powder

1/4 tsp. red pepper flakes

salt and **black pepper**, to taste

1 cup red **kidney beans**, cooked, drained and rinsed

1 cup **white kidney** beans, cooked, drained and rinsed

1 cup **black beans,** cooked drained and rinsed

1 cup great **Northern beans**, cooked, drained and rinsed

1 cup canned **corn kernel**s, drained and rinsed

2 1/2 cups **water**

2 tsp. dried **oregano**

2 tsp. dried **basil**

4 squares (75-percent) **chocolate, organic**

1 (28-oz.) can tomatoes

Juice of 1 lime Juice **of 1 lemon**

Into a Dutch oven, heat olive oil over medium heat; Mix in carrot onion, and bell pepper, and stri-fry until the onion becomes tender and translucent. Mix in red pepper flakes, chilli powder, and cumin seeds. Sprinkle salt and pepper to taste.

Put cover and cook over low heat for about 10 minutes, with stirring. Add the remaining ingredients, mix to blend, cover and simmer for about 20 minutes. Serve at once.

Amount Per Serving: Calories 396; Total Fat 139 g; Saturated Fat 4 g; Cholesterol 117.9 mg; Sodium 890.3 mg; Total Carbohydrate 63 g; Dietary Fiber 15 g; Iron 7 mg; Calcium 197 mg; Sugars 20.0 g; Protein 14

Healthier Fettuccine Alfredo

Meat out; tofu in. Cheddar Cheese out; nutritional yeast in. Margarine out; coconut butter in.

Makes 8 servings

1 1/2 lbs. extra firm **tofu,**

1/2 cup **vegetable broth**, Low salt

2 tsp. basil

1 tsp. onion powder

1/2 cup nutritional yeast

4 tbsp. coconut butter

Salt and pepper to taste

16 oz. fettuccine pasta

Into a pot of boiling lightly salted water, cook pasta for about 12 minutes or until al dente. Drain into a colander, rinse with running water and set aside on a bowl.

Into a food processor, combine the rest of the ingredients, process until smooth. Pour sauce over the pasta, toss to coat well. Season with some salt and pepper, and serve at once.

Amount Per Serving: Calories 241.9; Calories from Fat 25; Total Fat 2.8 g; Saturated Fat 0.4 g; Cholesterol 42.9

mg; Sodium 105.0 mg; Total Carbohydrate 38.2 g; Dietary Fiber 3.2 g; Sugars 0.3 g; Protein 17.5 g

Un-fried Fried Chicken

Deep- frying out; baking in

Makes 8 servings

6 (2 1/2-oz.) skinless boneless **chicken thighs**

6 boneless, skinless **chicken breast,** halved

2 large **limes**, halved

1/2 cup plain **non-fat** yogurt

3 cloves **garlic**, minced

2 tbsp. **cilantro,** chopped

1 **jalapeño**, halved, seeded, and chopped finely

1 cup **panko** breadcrumbs

1 tbsp. granulated **onion**

1 tsp. **salt**

1 tsp. ground **cumin**

1 tsp. chipotle **chili powder**

1 tsp. **paprika**

Preheat the oven to 375 ºF. Set a greased large wire rack on top of tin foil-lined baking pan.

Create pokes all over the chicken parts, drizzle lime juice and massage to ensure maximum blending. Into a small bowl, mix yogurt, with jalapeño, cilantro, and garlic. Pour into the chicken, mix well to blend. Set aside for about 10 minutes for flavour to develop.

Onto a large platter, mix breadcrumbs, with the rest of the seasonings. Coat chicken parts with this mixture and place on the prepared rack. Bake for about 25 minutes, turning once, or until golden brown and juicy.

Amount Per Serving: Calories 410; Total Fat 14 g; Saturated Fat 3 g; Cholesterol 166 mg; Sodium 869 mg; Total Carbohydrate 20 g; Dietary Fiber 1.0 g; Sugars 11 g; Protein 49 g

Quinoa Side Dish

Quinoa in; rice out

Makes 4 servings

1 tbsp. olive oil

1 cup uncooked quinoa

2 cups low sodium **vegetable broth**

2 tsp. **garlic,** chopped, lightly toasted

2 tbsp. **fresh parsley,** chopped

1/2 tbsp. **fresh thyme,** chopped

1/4 tsp. **salt**

1 small **onion**, finely chopped

1 dash fresh **lemon juice**

Into a saucepan, heat oil over medium flame. Cook quinoa, for about 5 minutes with stirring or until nicely toasted. Pour in broth, cover and bring to a boil. Reduce heat and simmer for about 15 minutes or until tender.

Meanwhile, into a non-stick pan, cook garlic and onions over medium flame for about 3 minutes or until garlic is lightly browned and onions, slightly tender.

Transfer cooked quinoa into a bowl, add the garlic, onions and herbs, sprinkle with salt and toss to blend.

Amount Per Serving: Calories 207; Total Fat 5.8 g; Cholesterol 8 mg; Sodium 300 mg; Total Carbohydrate 32 g; Dietary Fiber 3.9 g; Protein 6.9 g

Healthier Chicken Macaroni Salad

Heavy cream out; low-fat dairy and vegetable puree in

Makes 4 Servings

1 (6-oz.) box whole-grain **macaroni and cheese**

1/4 cup low-fat milk

2 tbsp. barbecue sauce

6 tbsp. sweet potato purée

1/2 cup **cooked chicken**, diced

Into a pot of boiling water, cook pasta for about 15 minutes or until al dente. Drain into a colander, rinse with running water and transfer into a bowl.

Into the same pot, combine milk, barbecue sauce, and sweet potato purée and bring to a simmer, stirring until well blended. Mix in the cooked chicken and macaroni, heat for about a minute or until heated through.

Amount Per Serving: Calories 116; Total Fat 4 g; Saturated Fat 2 g; Cholesterol 18 mg; Sodium 222 mg; Total Carbohydrate 12 g; Dietary Fiber 1.0 g; Sugars 4 g; Protein 7 g

Apple Nut Cereal

Oatmeal, quinoa, skimmed milk, apples and nuts are all in.

Makes 1 serving

1/4 cup **water**

1/4 cup skim milk

1 tbsp. **quinoa**

1/2 small **banana,** sliced

1 1/2 tbsp. rolled oats

1 tbsp. oat bran

1 pinch **salt**

1 pinch ground **cinnamon**

1 tbsp. **walnuts,** chopped

1 tsp. brown sugar

1/4 tsp. vanilla extract

Into a saucepan, combine milk and quinoa and boil over medium heat. Reduce heat to simmer for about 5 minutes or until quinoa just softens. Add the apples, oat bran, rolled oats, cinnamon and salt; cook with stirring for about 3 minutes or until thickened.

Place into a bowl; add nuts, sugar and vanilla. Mix and enjoy.

Amount Per Serving: Calories 220; Total Fat 6 g; Saturated Fat 2 g; Cholesterol 1 mg; Sodium 418 mg; Total Carbohydrate 37 g; Dietary Fiber 4.8 g; Protein 7 g

Zucchini Ribbons with Goat Cheese

Wheat pasta out; Zucchini Ribbons in

Makes 4 servings

1 tbsp. olive oil

1 tbsp. unsalted butter

1/4 cup **shallot**, finely minced

1 clove **garlic**, finely mince

1/2 tsp. crushed **red pepper flakes**

1/2 cup chicken broth

2 large **zucchinis,** seeded (about 4 cups)

1/4 cup **basil leaves** thinly sliced

2 1/2 oz. **goat cheese**, crumbled

salt and **pepper** to taste

Use a vegetable peeler to sliced zucchini into long ribbons.

Into a pan, heat olive oil and butter over medium flame; cook and stir the shallot for about 5 minutes until softened. Mix in garlic and red pepper flakes; cook and stir for about 3 more minutes until garlic softens.

Add in the chicken broth and zucchini ribbons, and cook, with light stirring for about 4 minutes, or until it boils and the zucchini strips are just tender. Put off the heat, sprinkle salt and pepper to taste.

Serve with basil leaves and crumbled goat cheese on top.

Amount Per Serving: Calories 155; Total Fat 12 g; Cholesterol 22 mg; Sodium 206 mg; Total Carbohydrate 8g; Dietary Fiber 2 g; Protein 6.2 g

Healthier Tomato Soup

Heavy cream, regular chicken broth out; 2% milk, low-sodium chicken broth in.

Makes 16 servings

4 cups low-sodium **chicken broth**

1 tbsp. sodium-free **margarine**

1 cup **tomatoes**, diced

4 cups reduced-sodium **tomato juice**

2 large **potatoes**, diced

1 large **onion**, diced

1/2 cup 2% low-fat milk

Salt and **pepper** to taste

Into a large saucepan, bring chicken broth and margarine to a boil over medium high flame. Add potatoes and boil. Reduce heat and simmer, covered for about 15 minutes or until potatoes are tender. Add tomatoes, and juice and continue simmering for about 5 minutes. Put off heat and using an immersion blender, blend the mixture until smooth.

Mix in milk and seasonings. Serve on individual serving bowls.

Amount Per Serving: Calories 67.9; Calories from Fat 12; Total Fat 0.1 g; Saturated Fat 0.0 g; Cholesterol 0.0 mg; Sodium 53.9 mg; Total Carbohydrate 15.4 g; Dietary Fiber 2.1 g; Sugars 5.9 g; Protein 2.0 g

Cauliflower "Rice"

White rice out, cauliflower in. Butter out; coconut oil in

Makes 4 servings

1 head **cauliflower**, cut into florets

1 tbsp. **water**

1 **lime**, juiced and zested

1/2 cup **cilantro**, chopped

2 tbsp. coconut oil

Put cauliflower florets into a blender and pulse until finely chopped. Transfer into a microwavable bowl and cook on high for about 7 minutes or until tender.

Add in the rest of the ingredients, toss until well blended.

Amount Per Serving: Calories 93; Total Fat 6 g; Cholesterol 15.0 mg; Sodium 87 mg; Total Carbohydrate 9.6 g; Dietary Fiber 4.2 g; Protein 3.1 g

Graham Cracker Pie Crust

Whole wheat crust out, Graham crackers crust in; Butter out, almond milk and coconut oil in

Makes 9 inch pie crust

1 1/2 cups crumbs of **Graham Crackers**

3 tbsp. coconut oil

3 tbsp. almond milk

Into a food processor, process crumbs until very fine. Gradually add oil and milk while processing into a crumbly mixture.

Spread mixture into a 9 inch pie pan and with firm fingers, push crumbs into the bottom and up the sides of the pan until it forms into a crust.

Use the pie crust for any bake or no bake pies of choice.

Amount Per Serving: Calories 300; Calories from Fat 150; Total Fat 17g; Saturated Fat 2.5g; Trans Fat

Cholesterol 15mg; Sodium 210mg; Potassium 75mg; Total Carbohydrate 36g; Dietary Fiber 1g; Sugars 17g; Protein 3g

Edamame Hummus

Chickpeas and Garbanzos out; Edamame in

Makes 4 servings

1/4 cup **tahini**

3 tbsp. lemon juice

1 **garlic clove**, peeled

2 tbsp. **fresh herbs** coarsely chopped (rosemary, thyme, and basil)

3 tbsp. **olive oil**

1/4 tsp. **salt** or to **taste**

Into a food processor, combine edamame, tahini, garlic, lemon juice, and fresh herbs; process until smooth. Drizzle olive oil while mixing oil is fully blended. Season with salt to taste. Enjoy as a side dish.

Amount Per Serving: Calories 150; Calories from Fat 110; Total Fat 12g; Saturated Fat 2g   ; Cholesterol 0 mg; Sodium 170mg; Potassium 170mg; Total Carbohydrate 6g; Dietary Fiber 2g; Sugars less than 1g;

Protein 5g

Herbed Turkey Wrap

Flour tortilla out, Lettuce wrap in

Makes 4 servings

2 tbsp. **olive** oil

1 **garlic** clove, minced

1/2 small **onion**, finely chopped

1/2 lb. ground **turkey**

2 tbsp. fresh **cilantro**

2 tbsp. lime juice

1/2 tbsp. fresh **ginger**, sliced

1 tsp. **cumin**

1 tsp. **pepper**

1 tsp. **salt**

1/8 cup **peanuts**, crushed

1 head **lettuce**

Into a pan, heat oil over medium high heat; sauté onions and garlic for about 3 minutes or until tender. Mix in ground turkey, cook and stir for about 5 minutes or until well cooked. Add the rest of the ingredients and coo for another 5 minutes.

Spread 1 large lettuce leaf. Spoon a large portion of turkey mixture into the centre and wrap over like a burrito. Make several wraps until all are used up.

Amount Per Serving: Calories 194.2; Calories from Fat 125; Total Fat 13.9 g; Saturated Fat 2.5 g; Cholesterol 44.8 mg; Sodium 662.7 mg; Total Carbohydrate 5.7 g; Dietary Fiber 1.9 g; Sugars 1.4 g; Protein 12.6 g

Healthier Egg Salad

Mayonnaise out; avocado mash in

Makes 2 servings

1 **avocado**, peeled, pitted, and mashed

3 **hard-boiled eggs**, peeled and chopped

1 tbsp. **sweet pickle** relish

1 tbsp. **onion,** chopped

1 tbsp. **celery,** chopped

1/2 tsp. balsamic vinegar

salt to taste

Into a bowl, combine avocado and eggs together; mix to blend. Add relish, onion, celery, vinegar and salt; mix well.

Amount Per Serving: Calories 289; Total Fat 22.7 g; Cholesterol 318 mg; Sodium 358 mg; Total Carbohydrate 12.6 g; Dietary Fiber 7 g; Protein 11.6 g

Healthier Meatloaf

Beef out; turkey in. Bread crumbs out; rolled oats in

Makes 4 servings

1 **egg**, beaten

1/4 cup low sodium **vegetable juice**

1/4 cup sour cream

1/2 tsp. ground black pepper

2 dashes hot pepper sauce

2 tbsp. Worcestershire sauce

1 tsp. dried **sage**

1 tsp. dried **parsley**

1 tsp. dried **oregano**

1 tsp. **salt**

 1/2 cup rolled oats

2 tbsp. **butter**

1/2 sweet **onion**, diced

1/2 green **bell pepper**, diced

2 stalks **celery**, diced

1 (16 oz.) can sliced **mushrooms**, drained

1 lb. ground turkey

1 (8 oz.) can **tomato sauce**

1/2 cup chili sauce

Preheat oven to 350 °F.

Into a bowl, combine the first 10 ingredients down to salt. Mix well to blend. Add oats, mix and set aside to soak.

Into a pan, heat butter over medium flame and sauté onions, bell peppers and celery for about 5 minutes or until tender. Transfer mixture into the bowl with oats. Add mushrooms and turkey and mix until well incorporated. Spread into a baking dish and top with a previously mixed tomato sauce and chilli sauce.

Bake for about an hour or until inner temperature reaches 165 ° F.

Amount Per Serving: Calories 405; Total Fat 19.9 g; Cholesterol 158 mg; Sodium 2083 mg; Total Carbohydrate 30.2 g; Dietary Fiber 6.1 g; Protein 30.2 g

Tofu Burgers

Tofu in; beef out

Makes 8 tofu patties

2 whole **eggs,** beaten

2 (16 oz.) packages **firm tofu,** drained

2 stalks **celery**, minced

1 small **onion**, minced

1 tbsp. **chili** powder

1 tbsp. ground **cumin**

1 tbsp. red curry paste

1 tbsp. **garlic,** minced

2 cups rolled oats

1 tbsp. coconut oil

Into a large bowl, whisk egg until smooth. Add the rest of the ingredients, except oil; mix thoroughly until well blended and tofu turn into small bits.

Form mixture into 8 patties.

Into a large non-stick pan, heat oil over medium heat; and cook patties for about 5 minutes per side or until crispy and golden brown.

Amount Per Serving: Calories 210; Total Fat 10.1 g; Cholesterol 53 mg; Sodium 83 mg; Total Carbohydrate 18.5 g; Dietary Fiber 3.1 g; Protein 13.9 g

Creamy Waffles with Strawberry Syrup

Heavy Cream out; cottage cheese in. Strawberry puree in; maple syrup out

Makes 6 waffles

4 tbsp. unsalted **butter**, melted

1 3/4 cups all-purpose flour

2 tsp. baking powder

1/4 tsp. baking soda

1/2 tsp. **salt**

1 cup cottage cheese

1 cup **milk**

2 large **eggs**

2 1/2 tbsp. **honey**

½ cup strawberry puree

Preheat a waffle iron.

Into a bowl, combine flour, salt, baking and powder baking soda. Mix well.

Into another bowl, whisk eggs with cottage cheese, milk and honey. Gradually pour into the flour mixture, mix until batter is formed. Mix in melted butter.

Lightly grease grids and scoop out 1/2 cup batter onto the hot iron. Evenly spread batter to the edge of the grids. Close and bake until golden brown.

Glaze with strawberry puree and serve.

Amount Per Serving: Calories 312.1; Calories from Fat 113; Total Fat 12.6 g; Saturated Fat 6.9 g; Cholesterol 94.0 mg; Sodium 540.3 mg; Total Carbohydrate 38.6 g; Dietary Fiber 1.0 g; Sugars 8.2 g; Protein 11.1 g

Kale Chips

Potato chips out; kale chips in

Makes 2 servings

1 bunch **kale**

1 tbsp. extra-virgin **olive oil**, divided

1 tbsp. balsamic vinegar

1 pinch **sea salt**, to taste

Preheat oven to 300 º F.

Trim kale by removing inner ribs. Tear leaves to 2-inch pieces wash in running water. Totally pat dry with paper towels.

Place torn kale leaves into a bowl, drizzle half of the oil; mix to fully coat. Add the rest of the oil, slowly mix until oil is well absorbed. Sprinkle vinegar and mix until fully coated. Spread the leaves evenly on a baking sheet and roast for about 20 minutes or until very crisp.

Serve after seasoning with salt.

Amount Per Serving: Calories 174; Total Fat 8.3 g;
Cholesterol 0 mg; Sodium 257 mg; Total Carbohydrate
22.5 g; Dietary Fiber 4.5 g; Protein 7.4 g

Banana Ice Cream

Heavy Cream out; banana puree in. Whole milk out, coconut milk in.

Makes 4 Servings

4 **bananas**, sliced

1/4 cup coconut milk

1 tsp. **vanilla**

Into a wax-paper-lined cookie pan, spread banana slices in single layer. Freeze for about 2 hours.

Into a food processor, place frozen banana slices and pulse several times until a course crumb texture is attained. Combine in milk and vanilla, process until a creamy smooth mixture is attained. Scrape once in a while the sides of the processor.

Transfer mixture into a freezer-safe container, cover and freeze for about 3 hours or until desired texture is attained.

Amount Per Serving: Calories 117.8; Calories from Fat 82; Total Fat 0.9 g; Saturated Fat 0.4 g; Cholesterol 2.1 mg; Sodium 8.7 mg; Total Carbohydrate 27.7 g; Dietary Fiber 3.0 g; Sugars 14.5 g; Protein 1.7 g

"Milk" Shake

Whole milk out; coconut cream in. Sugar out, fruit puree in.

Makes 2 Servings

1 cup coconut cream

1 very **ripe banana,** chopped

1 **peach**, peeled, cubed

1 cup **dates**

1 cup frozen **raspberries**

Into a food processor, combine cream, banana, peach and dates. Process until pureed. Add the raspberries, process until smooth but still tiny bits of berries are visible,

Serve in a tall glass or put in the freezer to chill.

Amount Per Serving: Calories 401.0; Calories from Fat 238; Total Fat 26.5 g; Saturated Fat 23.3 g; Cholesterol 0.0 mg; Sodium 75.2 mg; Total Carbohydrate 42.1 g; Dietary Fiber 7.5 g; Sugars 29.9 g; Protein 5.0 g

Penne with Arugula salad

Parmesan Cheese out, goat cheese in. Arugula in, iceberg lettuce out

Makes 6 servings

8 oz. penne pasta

1 cup **cherry tomatoes**, coarsely chopped

2 cups fresh **arugula**, chopped (stems included)

5 1/2 oz. **goat cheese**, crumbled

1/4 cup coconut oil

2 tsp. **garlic**, minced

1/2 tsp. each of **salt** and **black pepper**

Into a large pot of boiling salted water, cook pasta for about 15 minutes or until al dente. Drain into a colander, rinse with water and transfer into a bowl.

Into a mixing bowl, combine all other ingredients, mix until well blended. Combine with the pasta, toss to blend.

Amount Per Serving: Calories 317; Total Fat 26.5 g; Saturated Fat 23.3 g; Cholesterol 21 mg; Sodium 334 mg; Total Carbohydrate 29.7 g; Dietary Fiber 1.7 g; Protein 11 g

Gluten-Free Pan Cakes

Wheat flour out; Rice flour, potato starch and tapioca fours in.

Makes 10 pancakes

1 cup rice flour

3 tbsp. tapioca flour

1/3 cup potato starch

4 tbsp. dry buttermilk powder

1 packet **stevia**

1/2 tsp. baking soda

1/2 tsp. **salt**

1/2 tsp. xanthan gum

2 eggs

2 cups soy or coconut milk

Into a bowl, combine flours with the rest of the dry ingredients. Mix well to blend. Into another bowl, whisk eggs with milk. Gradually pour mixture into the dry mixture, mix until smooth batter is formed.

Into a large non-stick pan, heated over medium flame, scoop about tablespoonful portion of the batter, swirling to spread and cook until bubbly. Flip sides and cook for another minute until golden brown. ,

Serve immediately with fruit jams on top.

Amount Per Serving: Calories 147; Total Fat 5.8 g; Cholesterol 37 mg; Sodium 282 mg; Total Carbohydrate 20.4 g; Dietary Fiber 0.7 g; Protein 3.1 g

Healthier Brownies

Wheat flour out; coconut and almond flours in. Brown sugar out; muscovado sugar in.

Makes 12 brownies

3/4 cup brown **rice flour**

1/2 cup almond meal

3 tbsp. coconut flour

1 tsp. baking powder

1/2 tsp. **salt**

3/4 cup cocoa powder

3 tbsp. chia seed meal

1/2 cup plus 1 tbsp. **water**

1 cup Muscovado sugar

1/2 cup agave nectar

3 tbsp. **coconut but**ter

1 tsp. vanilla extract

Preheat oven to 350 ºF. Lightly grease a baking dish with coconut oil.

Into a bowl, combine flours and starch and the rest of the dry ingredients. Set aside.

Into a blender, soak chia meal with all the water for about 5 minutes. Add sugar and agave and at high speed until smooth. Add coconut butter and vanilla, blend to incorporate.

Pour mixture into the flour mixture, mix until smooth batter is formed. Spread into prepared dish and bake for about 50 minutes or until sides start to pull away from the dish. Cool on wire rack before cutting into desired slices.

Amount Per Serving: Calories 211; Total Fat 6.8 g; Cholesterol 0 mg; Sodium 188 mg; Total Carbohydrate 38.9 g; Dietary Fiber 4.1 g; Protein 3.1 g

Healthier Chocolate Chip Cookies

Sugar out; apple sauce in. Butter out; coconut oil in. Chocolate chips out, cocoa nibs in

Makes 3 dozen

3/4 cup **coconut oil**, melted

1/2 cup applesauce

1/2 cup packed **brown sugar**

1 egg

1 tsp. **vanilla** extract

1 1/4 cups all-purpose **flour**

1 cup graham cracker crumbs

1/2 tsp. **salt**

1/2 tsp. baking soda

3/4 cup milk chocolate pieces

2 cups cocoa nibs

1/2 cup **pecans**, roughly chopped

Preheat oven to 375 °F.

Into a bowl, whip coconut oil and applesauce until smooth. Add egg and vanilla, whip for another minute until fully blended. Into another bowl, combine flour, salt, baking soda and graham cracker crumbs. Mix well. Gradually mix this mixture into the wet mixture, until fully incorporated. Add chocolates and fold to blend.

Drop spoonful portions onto a baking sheet, pat to flatten and bake for about 9 minutes or until lightly browned. Cool a bit and transfer to a wire rack to cool totally.

Amount Per Serving: Calories 322; Total Fat 8.1 g; Cholesterol 33 mg; Sodium 195 mg; Total Carbohydrate 40.2 g; Dietary Fiber 2 g; Protein 3.1 g

Creamy Mussel and Shrimp Soup

Heavy cream out; fat-free half-and-half in

Makes 8 Servings

1 lb. live **mussels** in shells, washed, trimmed

12 oz. small **shrimp** in shells

1 cup **salt**

1 (14 oz.) can reduced-sodium **chicken broth**

1 tbsp. olive oil

1 cup **leeks**, finely chopped

2   cloves **garlic**, minced

1/8 tsp. ground **turmeric**

1/4 tsp. ground **black pepper**

1 cup fat-free **half-and-half**

1 tbsp. finely chopped **fresh basil**

Into a very large container, combine 8 cups of cold water and 5 tbsp. of the salt. Soak the mussels for about 15 minutes. Drain into a colander and rinse mussels. Repeat process two times more, using the same amounts of water and salt. Rinse well.

Into a large pot, boil chicken broth with 1-1/2 cups water over high heat. Add mussels, lower heat, cover and simmer for about 6 minutes or until shells are open and mussels are cooked throughout. Discard the unopened mussels. Add shrimp, at the last 3 minutes of cooking.

Cover a colander with cheesecloth and strain cooking liquid into a bowl. Place seafood into a bowl until cooled to handle. Set aside both.

Remove meat from mussels and peel and devein shrimp. Discard shells.

Into a large skillet, heat oil over medium flame; and cook leeks and garlic for about 4 minutes or until tender. Pour in reserved cooking liquid, saffron, and pepper and bring to a boil. Lower heat and gently boil uncovered for about 15 minutes. Mix in mussels, shrimps and half-and-half and heat further until heated through.

Sprinkle with basil and serve.

Amounts Per Serving: Calories 79, Fat, total (g) 4, Cholesterol (mg) 16, Saturated fat (g) 1, Carbohydrates (g) 7, fiber (g) 0, Protein (g) 3, Sodium (mg) 456,

Turkey Wrapped in Collard Greens

Flour tortillas out; collard greens in

Makes 4 Servings

1 large bunch **collard greens**

1 lb. lean ground turkey

3/4 tsp. **salt**

2 tsp. ground cumin

2 tsp. red chili pepper flakes

2 tsp. **onion** powder

1 tsp. **garlic** powder

1 tsp. dried **oregano**

1 cup enchilada sauce

Preheat oven to 400 º F.

Trim off thick stems of collard greens. Place into a steamer and steam for about 4 minutes or until just wilted. Set aside to cool.

Into a bowl, combine ground turkey and all of the seasonings. Mix well. Make 4 equal portions and form each into a mini log. Wrap each log with collard green leaves like a burrito.

Arrange wrap logs, seam side down into a baking dish. Spread some enchiladas on tops, cover dish with tin foil and bake for about 40 minutes or until cooked through.

Amount Per Serving: Calories 200.3; Calories from Fat 83; Total Fat 9.2 g; Saturated Fat 2.3 g; Cholesterol 78.2 mg; Sodium 915.6 mg; Total Carbohydrate 6.8 g; Dietary Fiber 1.9 g; Sugars 2.2 g; Protein 23.9 g.

Thanks!

That's all the recipes for now, I hope you liked them.

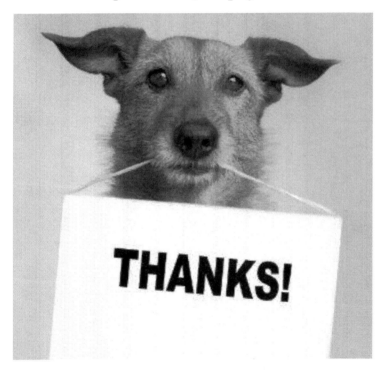

Finally, if you enjoyed this book, then I'd like to ask you for a favor, would you be kind enough to leave a review for this book on Amazon? It'd be greatly appreciated!

Click here to leave a review for this book on Amazon!

http://amzn.to/1tqrxpy

Thank you and good luck!

Don't Forget your Two FREE Bonuses:

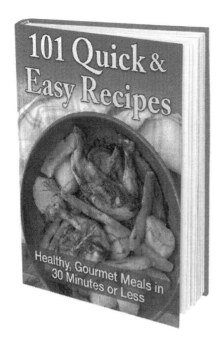

Do you waste your money on take-out because you don't have time to cook? Do you want more variety in your diet? Well this Recipe Book is for you!!!

"101 Quick & Easy Recipes" is the quickest and easiest way to create gourmet and great tasting meals all in 30 minutes or less! Inside this magnificent book, you'll get **101 Recipes** you'll absolutely love, all of which can be made quickly and easily... in 30 minutes or less!!

As a thank you, I want to give you this amazing collection of recipes, completely free of charge, as my gift to you. There is no catch... it's really free, I promise. Just click the link below to download it now!

Click here to get it FREE!!

http://bit.ly/free101recipes

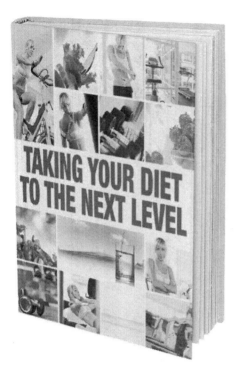

Do you want to lose weight, but nothing has worked long term? Do you have trouble changing your habits and end up falling back into the same unhealthy routine? Are you having trouble reaching the level of health and fitness success that you want to achieve? Well this Report is for you!!!

"Taking Your Diet to the Next Level" is an insightful report explaining why you aren't reaching the level of success that you want, and how to change that. It goes through each stage of dieting, weight loss and making healthy changes and provides strategies for how to break through those walls that are sopping you from achieving the diet, weight loss and fitness success that you deserve.

As a thank you, I want to give you this amazing report, completely free of charge, as my gift to you. There is no catch... it's really free, I promise. Just click the link below to download it now!

Click here to get it FREE!!

http://bit.ly/nextleveldiet

Check Out Some of My Other Books

Below you'll find some of my other popular books that are popular on Amazon and Kindle as well. Simply click on the links below to check them out.

Clean Eating: The only real way to be naturally skinny, lose weight, and have more energy than you can possibly imagine

Anti Inflammatory Diet: How to Fight Inflammation, Heart Disease and Chronic Pain just by Eating Delicious Food

If the links do not work, for whatever reason, you can simply search for these titles on the Amazon website to find them.

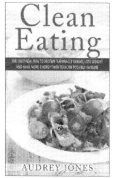
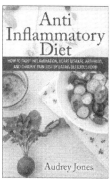

This document is geared towards providing exact and reliable information in regards to the topic and issue covered. The publication is sold with the idea that the publisher is not required to render accounting, officially permitted, or otherwise, qualified services. If advice is necessary, legal or professional, a practiced individual in the profession should be ordered.

- From a Declaration of Principles which was accepted and approved equally by a Committee of the American Bar Association and a Committee of Publishers and Associations.

The information provided herein is stated to be truthful and consistent, in that any liability, in terms of inattention or otherwise, by any usage or abuse of any policies, processes, or directions contained within is the solitary and utter responsibility of the recipient reader. Under no circumstances will any legal responsibility or

Made in the USA
Middletown, DE
20 May 2016